Yoga "Pretzel" Bliss

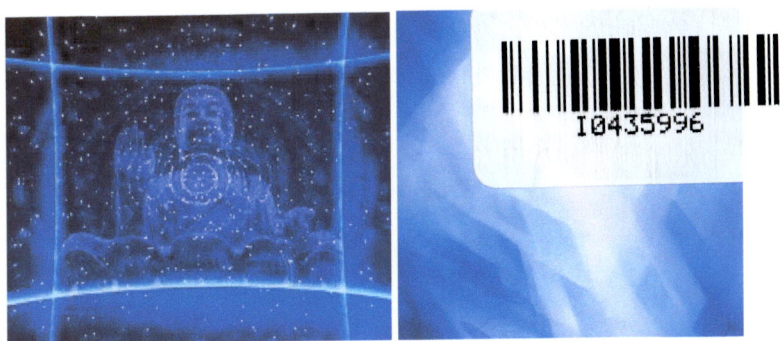

"Wifi Hot-Spot" Power Beyond Pose; Transforming Spine Pain into Paradise

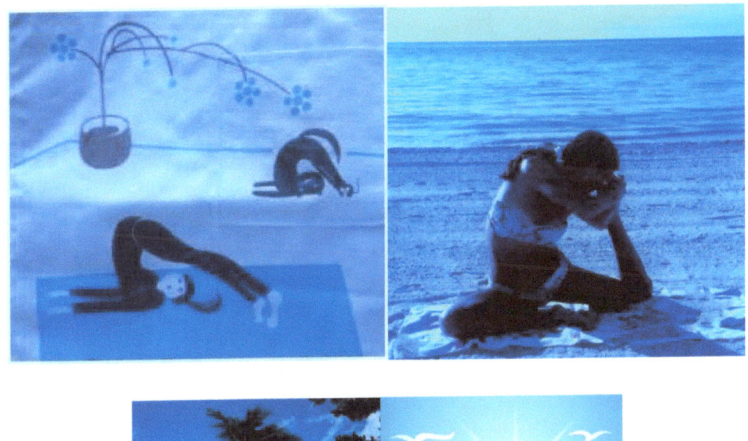

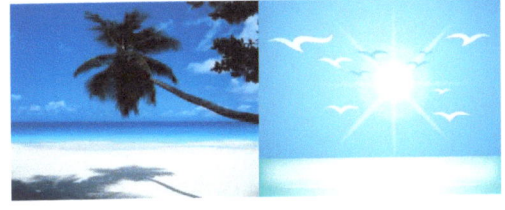

Maryann Fenicato, Esq., Ph.D.

DEDICATION

This is for all yoga lovers, full range from novice to natural.

Here's how to go far beyond its physical benefits, and turn even terrible spine problems into chi, prana "God goosebump" bliss.

Enjoy!

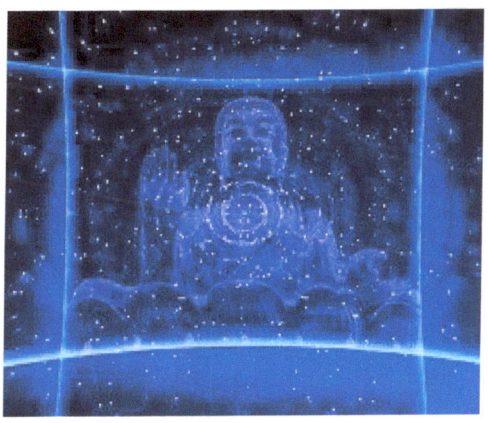

CONTENTS

ACKNOWLEDGMENTS

Above and beyond all of my usual acknowledgements, this time I must first thank the author of a yoga book I read long ago, so long I have forgotten her name and its title. Back then, all my spine problems had not yet manifested multifariously, so its basic hatha yoga poses fixed me up 'real quick and sparked a deep love, respect and humble gratitude for the practice that will never end.

On the other hand, I will never forget the beautiful, pretty light and airy pastel blue beach pictures, which may have done more for my soul than meets the eye. Perhaps they called me out to my destiny, signs amplifying a homing signal to Florida set off long before.

Accordingly, I also thank everyone and everything that did more for me than I ever could have initially understood or imagined, which hopefully this book will do, in turn, too, for all of you.

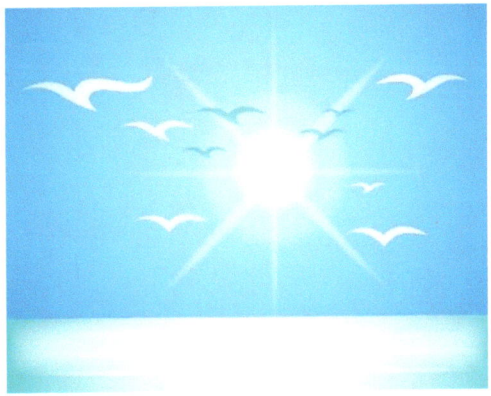

1
INTRODUCTION:
LIGHTHOUSE LANTERN

Yoga classes are supposed to help a person feel BETTER, right?

Ah, but what if certain injuries seem beyond help or hope, and jealous students make classes the opposite of a healing sanctuary?

Do you give up?

Heck no!

Why?

Because a "wifi" connection to ultimate aid is available anywhere, which can turn your painful "hot-spots" into pleasurable paradise.

This book will provide proof and explain how to tap in to chi or prana power beyond pose, connecting all the way up to nirvana.

In fact, your pain IS the transformative plane ticket to fly that high!

Why settle for mere physical benefits (think, for example, cold Pittsburgh) when this book could be your travel guide, this author your travel agent, to a tropical paradise (think Key West)—right?

In fact, the key is NOT to think too much, especially when balancing. Instead, for each pose, one must balance many things, your body and your mind, resting in the pose but not too much, as you accomplish it actively, holding on loosely, but not letting go.

That paradox point of active stillness IS the celestial "stargate," the crossing or crossover point. Finding and holding it without going over the physical edge taps the force source that takes you beyond.

Yet, before this book seems to blow too much sun shine or star light, patience is a requisite virtue, the positive side of karma. In other words, it may NOT happen the first time you try, and it may still may elude you however long thereafter. Cheaters never win, so just like karmic justice, there may be a prerequisite waiting period for each person to prove their "faith" or fortitude. In fact, it may happen when you least expect it, long after hope is lost.

But, when the time comes, it will blow through your problems, no matter what. When you're due, it will "get 'er done" for you.

So, to provide hope and inspiration for others, this book will also recount various unfortunate circumstances which could've caused even a big a fan of yoga like this author, to throw in the towel. These include physical complications stemming from two spine injuries to the same spot, which made various earlier injuries come back to haunt her, as if waking up the dead. Things got so bad at one point that the author suffered a terrible two tag-team: 1) sciatic STABBING pain in her left hip running down her entire left leg, and 2) EXCRUCIATING neck pain that actually felt worse when stretched, even during YOGA! Believe it or not, it was as if yoga had turned against her, too, because for a long period of time, no stretch worked unless pulled or taken far past difficult poses, where pain then came from the other side—no way out or any relief!

Having studied yoga herself at home, the answer seemed to be to take a class with others, when she could ask the teacher various questions. However, when it became clear to her that nothing but one particular very difficult "pretzel" twist often shown on magazine covers would ease her pain, although the teacher quickly helped and showed her how, the students became jealous. Thus, before achieving any effective healing, she "walked away" from an initially sweet sanctuary that suddenly went over to the dark side.

Yet, despite the continued pain, she never gave up practicing on her own, and one day, when she least expected it, the "spirit" moved her into an even more difficult position, which worked wonders. Done once a day, following non-local assistance, ever since she's "walked away" and said "good bye" to all chiropractors!

Lighting the way like a caring lighthouse or angelic lantern, this book will fully explain, yet take you beyond that, and more. Enjoy!

2
LET'S GET PHYSICAL!

That silly eighties song has long-been burned into my brain, but just like the chapter in my carb "diet" way-of-life book, this title truly fits this one just as perfectly, both good and bad.

Why?

A. Physical Triggers

Unfortunately, many people try yoga only after they have to, because of a physical injury. Others, may see it as a great workout, so, especially those pressed for time, may skip the "prayers," going straight for the calorie-burning physically challenging classes.

Yet, although that's absolutely correct, there's so much more, many other options available, that can go deeper and work wonders.

B. Simple Stretches

On the other hand, simple stretches can accomplish more than the difficult "pretzel" poses, so the right attitude is key.

So, let's start at the beginning and go on from there.

C. Basic Classes Versus Self Study

Although class teachers can show you the right way, many beginner students may shy away, assuming that other students will know more, make then look bad, or even laugh, if they don't get it or pick it up quick. Everyone, however, had to start somewhere, even those who seem to be natural yogis. Since private lessons might be costly, otherwise impractical or impossible, another answer is home school or self-study. Although you may only have a book to help you, you'd have pictures to go on, and your own body to check in with, the ultimate judge as to what feels good or works for you.

So, with those pros and cons in mind, judge that, too.

Another idea would be to do both, the best of both worlds.

But, if you get hooked, the best way might be books and research, which will allow you to excel far past scheduled classes.

D. Quick Fix Elixir

Yoga could be as swift as knockout karma, packing quite a punch. It could be love at first "sight," that is, of course, the first pose or stretch that suddenly tanks or rocks your world. A long-held pain could quickly disappear, become a "done deal," never to return. No wonder one could easily get hooked on such a quick fix elixir.

E. Basic Poses—Easy Stretches

If you have one typical pain or problem, especially if it has not lasted too long, you are young, and it has not been complicated or exacerbated by other problems, a basic pose or could do the trick. The key might be to see them as easy stretches with fun challenge.

F. Diagnosing Difficult Problems with Extremes

But, if you have a difficult problem, such as a second injury in the same place, that's been compounded by many other injuries, not to mention your age, etc., to find a good fix or lasting relief, you may have to kick it up.   In cases of terrible pain, however, people may not want to wait or play it safe, so they may seek extremes.

G. Ashtanga Yoga

Ashtanga yoga is one of the more rapid extremes, going straight for the physical burn and benefits, right out of the gate. Most classes skip more than initial prayers, centering and stretches, starting out standing, etc. These can be great workouts, but the reason they seem exciting is much more than the adrenaline rush between poses. Since many poses are done rather quickly, each taps various muscle groups, the quantity of which can make you feel good all over. But, working out a difficult pain may require something else.

H. Lyenger Yoga

Lyenger yoga is perhaps ashtanga's opposite extreme, so slow. If ashtanga were the proverbial hare, this would indeed be the turtle. It holds poses much longer than typical classes, possibly too long. Since only a few basic poses would be held, give it a good try, but know that it may not work, either.

I. The Golden Mean Between Extremes

The "Golden Mean" between extremes is an oldie, but a goodie, wise advice first imparted by Ancient Greek philosopher Aristotle and many others since, tried and true that has withstood the test of time. It's founded on, or otherwise arrives at, just plain common sense, suggesting moderation rather than extremes. But, since many kinds of yoga and an infinite number of poses might fall into a such a wise, moderate category, how should one choose?

J. Trial and "Error"

Perhaps the most effective sage, scientific way to choose would be trial and error, also known as "process of elimination." This is even more true with yoga, since just about any pose tried would be beneficial to some extent, no regrettable error. One simply keeps trying until one finds success. But, what if it still eludes you? Should one sample different poses or more difficult variations?

K. Matching Fire with Fire

If a physical problem is difficult, it stands to reason that its solution may be equal, so one might have to exceed the otherwise wise (ha!) limits of moderation. One might have to match fire with fire.

L. Gut/God/Grace

Regardless of elusiveness, there is always an answer. Even logic includes one good (ha!) illogical (ha!) axiom—when there is no logical answer, the answer IS illogical. Since yoga is already past western medicine, and other eastern modalities (acupuncture, massage, reiki, as well as color, smell or shop (ha!) therapy, etc.) may not have worked either, one may have to go into the great beyond. Luckily, however, it is easy to "go there" with just one's gut feeling, which is not merely emotional, rather, God or grace. Although it took time, that's what finally worked for this author.

M. "I Just Knew"

Several times, this author noticed a pose and asked the teacher to be taught. Each time, she humbly explained that she only wanted to learn because she was sure it would help her spine problems, so the teachers showed her immediately. Unfortunately, the first few only helped to a certain extent, so this author kept looking. Then, one day, she saw "it," eka pada rajakapotasana, aka "one legged pigeon pose," done as follows on the cover of a yoga magazine:

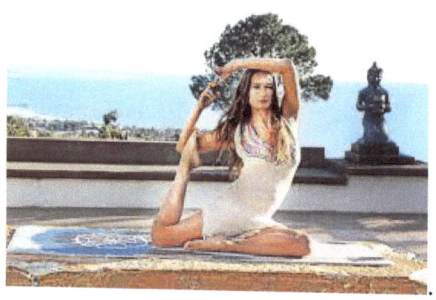

Immediately, she "just knew" that was it.

Although it turned out to be the one, things suddenly got nasty.

Here's why:

N. Cover Girl Jealousy

The other students had been jealous for a while, that is, also of the all the attention this author had been getting. Seeing her do this "cover shot" took them over the edge to the dark side. The ring leader used to be "queen bee" at some other yoga place, but this was far beyond anything she could do or fathom. But, the bigger problem is island-wide here in Key West, namely, people here expect newcomers to pale in comparison, and they get especially jealous of anything that seems to come easy for others, assuming they never worked hard many long years to get up to it. So, although it was a yoga class, the other students as well as some of the teachers were easy kindle for her to light a fire under once the owner left. Soon, it turned from a nice, close sanctuary into an unhealthy snake pit with a snarling lynch mob. Since even the other teachers did a Dr. Jekyll and Mr. Hyde, and this author would only wind up getting hurt even more, she got her money back and walked away. Now she's very glad she did.

Here's why:

O. Worse Curse

After that, things got worse in almost every area of her life, so bad, in fact, that this author felt cursed. In particular, and most relevant to this, although she did not know their reasons at the time, mean, jealous people all over the island also gave this author dirty looks, thinking she was faking her pain for attention. They assumed that anyone who could do any back bend must be ok—how stupid!

Eventually, however, the PHYSICAL pain caused her to do something dire, travel far away seeking a cure.

P. The Cure

But, in so doing, she not only faced her fears and fried the curse, but also stepped up to her destiny, and got rewarded in many ways.

Specifically, she eventually found a practitioner who actually helped her more than any chiropractor, either out of the goodness of his heart or because he couldn't fake it and milk her money each week—right? Afterward, she also had no choice but to move a very heavy piece of luggage in the opposite direction that she normally does, that sealed what he did into place—how about that?

Thus, once she returned, she resumed doing yoga, tentatively and painfully at first, but once she began writing these books, the real problem, the biggest and most important one of all, the pain lessened and she eventually found a more difficult permutation of that pose that holds her hips in place and make her neck pain more manageable all day. Here's the cure:

This is a picture of that same pose, now done in the opposite direction, twisting backward skillfully, toe touching the "third eye:"

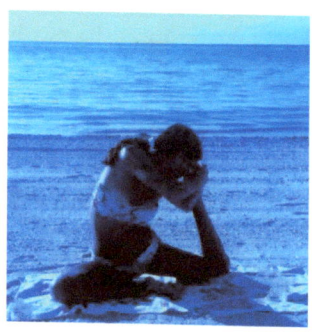

Q. Cover this!

Now turning such past bitter lemons into sweet lemonade, it now one of the nice pictures on the COVER of THIS book, which instantaneously proves them wrong per se, since it will obviously be used for altruistic reasons, to help anyone all over the world.

R. Emotional Pain Pockets, Etc.

Yet, even the physical aspects of yoga simultaneously tap much deeper things. For instance, certain poses, especially those never before tried, can release pockets of emotional pain, as well.

S. Focus Shift

Since there is, indeed, far more to get from yoga than just physical, this book will next shift its focus to the greatest of these, the very best thing of all, believe it or not, LOVE!

3
LOVIN' THE "PRETZEL" OVEN

A. Love Boat

What could make a person fall in love at first "sight" with yoga?

Instead of a slow boat, what could take them to paradise so fast?

Is the answer just physical or even emotional pain pocket release?

Could it possibly be trippin' or happily tapping into past lives?

B. All the Way

Even if the answer is a past life, during that life, to reach its blissful joy, one would have to go deeper, loving it and yet letting go, all the way to paradise, to God, to Love, itself.

C. Reuniting with LOVE

If people do not want to "go there," believe it's possible, one of the biggest hold ups is what they may have been taught about God.

Although life is often hard and unfair, there are many answers out these, proving that God may not be fearsome fire and brimstone, watching us from on high to punish out sins—notice how easily that concept could be misused to discipline children with fear, which can in turn, easily backfire. How could that continue if Jesus taught us that God IS love? Here's how: He paid for that teaching with his life. After he died, who knows how much of his teachings and even the Bible was severely edited, changed, omitted or otherwise altered to fit the secretive power-tripping agendas of male patriarchs, especially those wielding high church positions. Today, more and more proof is coming out, about all sorts of related things, especially how the Divine Feminine was denigrated, helping us to finally go back to the way it was meant to be, LOVE.

For eons before that, all over the globe, "She" was worshipped in various forms, eventually Christianized and replaced by St. Mary, who was mostly reduced to being nothing more than Jesus' mere Mother. Then, for centuries, any woman who did not, for instance, cower down to men, etc., could have been hunted down as a witch and burned at the stake to take and usurp all power from women.

Jesus taught a balance between the two, but since he was such a charismatic leader, men abused his power and killed him to take it.

Thus, to get more out of yoga, and ideally balance our whole lives, let alone yoga poses, is by going back to reunite with that LOVE.

D. Bliss This!

Best of all, there's no need to limit this LOVE. We can take it all the way to bliss, nirvana. Why? Remember, even the Bible says we were meant to live in the Garden of Eden, beautiful total paradise. Unlike many of our real parents (sigh!), that's what our benevolent, supernatural God gave us and wanted us to enjoy, evermore. Most importantly, we must thus realize that this bliss is our natural state, our spiritual home on high, so we can go there anytime we want!

E. Been There, Done That

If such extreme bliss seems impossible, this book will prove you've already been there, done that. In fact, it is so easy, you may miss it, but only because you may not realize WHAT it is.

F. How Sweet it is

Unfortunately, most people get there in bad ways that can have terrible consequences, i.e., smoking, drinking, sex, drugs and rock and roll. If you're surprised that smoking is in that list, don't be, because it proves the next point. Even something as seemingly small alters your state of consciousness to some extent, then your emotions, the rest of your body, etc., follow and adjust as well-- notice how much better that is for smokers. But, good, sweet stuff is even BETTER than that, because it's much easier and quicker, and once cultivated, it can take you as far out as LOVE itself.

G. Been There, Done That!

Although you've done stuff like this countless times, perhaps never realizing the underlying awesome power, let's try it. Think of something so sweet, nice, etc., which may be different for everyone, that sweeps you off your feet, wafts you up to seventh heaven the very minute you think about it. It could be a sunset or sunrise, a picture of your guy, girl husband, wife, child, grandchild, car, boat, summer house, and the list goes on—see? It can include imagining things, fantasizing or even daydreaming. Reading books can zone you out and watching movies can literally move you in many ways. If only for a moment, it takes you out and away from, your real life problems, then you've "been there, done that."

D. In the Zone

Now, let's take it one step further. Such bliss is NOT limited to things that are sweet, silent or sedentary. All kinds of movement, from slow meditative seemingly boring sweeping to wonderful, exciting "what a feeling" dancers, and even gold medal Olympians or rugged football athletes, etc., know how to get into the "zone." The latter are opposite extremes, so let's take it back down a notch.

E. Moving Meditation—Powerful Payoff

Yoga is, in fact, a balancing act, quite like a Golden Mean in between those extremes. To accomplish most poses, one must literally learn to hang on the "edge," a paradox point of active rest. Although walking and other forms of easier moving meditation exist, yoga's got that challenge, and bliss is its full potential payoff.

'Gotta love that!

F. Seeing the Key

The right ATTITUDE is key.

G. Trying too Hard

Just like a romantic suitor trying to hard could get rebuffed, the same is true with yoga.

H. More than Physical Skill

A person could do a pose perfectly, but never feel any bliss. Another could barely try and quickly win such a "power ball lottery." Why? Because it takes much more than physical skill.

I. When the Dancer Becomes the Dance

Today, we can watch many 'wanna be dancers and vocalists on TV. Many may have skill, but few will "have something"—gee, what could that be? We know it when we see or hear it—it moves us beyond, as well. If so, what really happened is that the performer let go and went past us into the zone, enjoying it so much that our soul could melt, we could be swept off our feet and taken along for the ride. It's when the dancer stops thinking about anything, steps, music, crowd, judges, etc., and lets the dance itself take over.

J. That's What LOVE IS!

If one could feel that lovin' feeling, not lose it, during yoga in general, but especially at the cross over points, resting in the pose yet enjoying the exciting challenge, bingo! That's what LOVE is.

K. The Icing on the Cake

As if that were not enough, above and beyond lessening, relieving or eliminating pain, continued practice could actually transform terrible pain into sheer "God-goosebump" bliss. It's like icing on the cake, which you get to have and eat it, too. It is not, however, guaranteed to all, and spiritual prerequisites do exist.

L. Quality Time

I recall a relevant song lyric which can be paraphrased as follows: a person must "put in the QT for the booty." It means that quality time must be spent for relationships to work. That is so true for yoga. Time is needed to understand and be able to do the poses in the first place, of course, but to hit the bliss button, even more must be added. God wants a relationship with each of us—He wants us to spend time with Him. Thus, how much will depend on each person, because He, chi or prana can see inside your heart.

M. No Expectations

Neither nirvana or pain relief during yoga can be forced or expected. In fact, it is more likely to happen when least expected.

N. Let Go and Let God

Since basic hatha yoga poses suddenly and permanently fixed an earlier problem long ago, this author thought it would happen again, but by then, too many injuries had been sustained for quick, total relief. In fact, for a long time, the harder she tried, the worse it became, because stretching too far caused pain on the other side. It was only after she let go of that expectation, learned to live with the pain for a while, that things started to change. Instead, change was required elsewhere, in her case, the writing of these helpful books. After her fifth, something released on another level, and long after she ever expected to feel bliss again during yoga, it suddenly returned sweetly on its own, quite like a writing reward. By then, the twist she came up with for one legged king pigeon pose served as a wonderful anchor, sustaining terrible pain relief throughout the day. Although she is never fully free of pain, she has certainly said "good bye" to all chiropractors. Thus, this story demonstrates that the key was, indeed, to let go and let God.

O. Others' Advice, Especially Chiropractor's!

Another prerequisite is to free oneself from advice from others, who may have their own agendas to lead you astray, especially chiropractors! This author's pain used to be so bad that it returned right after chiropractor visits, before even getting to the elevator! Upon consultation, she was told all sorts of conflicting things, which steered her away from healing and gee, let's guess, towards more costly visits—right? Once drinking Diet Coke was targeted, preposterously, this author became determined to free herself from them permanently, but said nothing until she found her own cure. Eventually, she stopped going altogether, and received a call saying it had been too long since her last visit. When she replied that she had no plans to ever return, but have a nice day, they were stunned.

Oh, well!

P. Freely Open

Once free from one's own expectations and others' advice, the key is to remain or be freely open, and not just during yoga. This author used to have no idea what that meant, either, OK, but hindsight has revealed that we really are better off being open to His will, not ours, and we really must thank God for unanswered prayers. So, one way to remain freely open is to recall various times in our lives when things got much better once we did let go and let God. Such sweet memories are the ticket.

Q. Soar on Sweetness

But, why stop there! Why not get there even quicker and easier as already mentioned by contemplating whatever moves or melts your heart and soul. Why not open the celestial sweet door and soar!

R. Lovin' the Oven

Since pain can remain, regardless, however, another key is to see it as a ticket to paradise. Bread has to cook in an oven before it is done, so we may have to enjoy the journey, not arrive immediately. Eventually transformed, if one has patience, never gives up, puts in the quality time, and is willing to wait for His will, such an initially painful oven door can become a blissful heavenly stargate. Ahhhh!

S. Back to the Future

To shed an even brighter lighthouse, lantern, qualitative light on such an optimum connection, this book will now go back to the future, discussing it from various related perspectives, ranging from ancient practices to modern technology.

4
BACK TO THE FUTURE

A. Definition

Yoga comes from the Sanskrit root *yuj*, which means "to join" or "to yoke." As to what it seeks unity with, answers include all sorts of good stuff, God, Gaia, Light, Spirit, etc.

B. Method

The method by which a person could achieve or arrive at such union itself requires a unity, that is, body, mind and soul. Physical postures alone could not cut it. One would also need a proper or pure intention, and a balancing of various other factors.

C. Strike a Pose

The poses themselves, however, are a powerful combination of muscle groups, etc. Yet, one can easily go beyond, because the latent potential of each is like a dial up connection with the Divine.

D. Ecstatic Poses

If "dial up" seems dated, that was done on purpose, because many other related practices have been done for eons. Among those most similar are "ecstatic poses, " which can be done for many reasons. In her first book entitled, "Ecstatic Body Postures: An Alternate Reality Workbook," author Belinda Gore explains where and how they were discovered after all these years, namely, all over the world, from statues found in sacred places, etc. It lists and categorizes them according to various purposes, including healing, divination and spirit journeys. Her second book, "The Ecstatic Experience: Healing Postures for Spirit Journeys," provides more.

E. Electronic Age

As time moved on into modernity, one could use lots of electronic objects as metaphors, such as radio antennas, television "rabbit ears," satellite dishes, etc. Notice they are also, yet seemingly more scientifically, such as math equations, configured, strategized and purposefully set up to receive a specific frequency, signal, etc.

F. Latest Computer Technology

Today, high speed internet connection is all the rage. Lots of options are available, with "Wifi" hot-spots topping the list. But, despite the technology, the concept is still the same—configuring physical objects, passwords and enhancements according to certain precise specifications past-proven to provide desired results.

G. Religious Magic

Notice that religious rituals and magic spells or incantations are similar, although aiming higher and farther beyond. Again, physical items are strategically positioned and/or utilized in specific ways, and combined with other equally important things, such as preset words, passwords, prayers, spells, etc.

H. Science or Spiritual

In the past, both were the same. Today, where one would draw the line between them is hard to say. Scientists used to think the world was flat, airplanes foolish, etc. Thus, it's ever-changing and illusive.

I. Food & Drink Recipes

For those of you who prefer day-to-day examples, note that recipes are analogous, yet down to earth concepts, that also begin with basic physical ingredients, embellished with other items like spices, but the most important one of all is the "wavelength" or skill of the cook or bartender. Anyone can cook, but will it be worth it? The best ones do what they love and love what they do, thus they also add intangibles like love.

J. Pick Your Pleasure

This "back to the future" list could continue. Those provided, however, are plenty, from which anyone could pick their pleasure, their cup of tea. They are all nothing but specific examples of the same bottom line: It's EASY to go beyond to bliss.

K. Pretzel Poses

Difficult or even potentially dangerous "pretzel" poses are NOT necessary. Although they are really worth doing for other reasons, basic poses and simple stretches can dial up the Divine if your heart and soul is in the right place, etc.

L. Overall Combo

A challenging pose can relieve or manage physical pain. But, a spiritual "wifi" hot-spot is not accomplished with just one thing, even a seemingly perfect pose, rather, but an overall combination.

M. Proper Intent

A karmic waiting period may be imposed to produce a proper intent. Wanting too much too soon will not work. Being willing to wait on God's will is the answer.

N. Soaring Spirit

Yet, the best thing of all is a soaring spirit that knows no limit as to how high it can fly. As depicted in Disney movies, one must BELIEVE they can fly (and touch the sky) before they can or will.

O. Trusting THE Spirit

Most important, however, is trusting the Great Spirit, God, chi, prana, universal or cosmic energy, or whatever else you call it, to move you. In fact, it may not just move you to nirvana, but the chicken could come before the egg—it could move you into a pose variation that really relieves you pain and does that, as well.

P. The Secret Secret

Yet, the secret to that may be secret, hence the next chapter...

Q. Love's Got Everything to Do With It!

But, before we move on to that, the reason the title of this chapter was, "Lovin' the Pretzel Oven," is because unlike Tina Turner's song, love does have everything to do with this. To amplify that visually, here's a picture of a heart-shaped angel. This one was chosen because it is purposefully out of focus, leaving the possible or potential details up too your imagination. Enjoy.

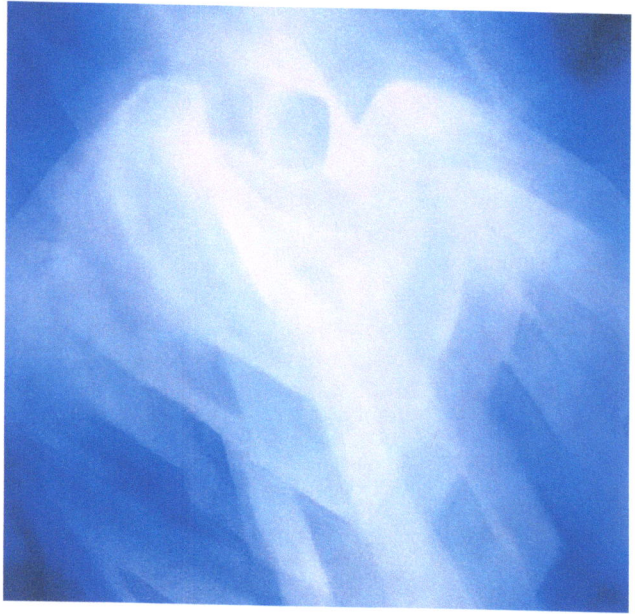

5
THE SECRET SECRET

A. The "Snarl"

If it seemed impossible that a healing yoga studio could switch from a sanctuary into a living hell, get a load of this second true story concerning a teacher. It's the last thing one would expect.

In order to do proper research for this book, this author recently went to a different studio, thinking she already knew the teacher. He turned out to be someone else, and something else, entirely.

Since she purposefully went a few minutes before a scheduled class end to watch a little while, he did greet her and ask if he could help. However, when she politely and humbly indicated, out of respect for all the students, that she'd wait until after class was over, he seemed to purposefully delay class by over fifteen minutes. She also thought she saw a sinister grin, as if he was enjoying making her wait, but dismissed it in her mind—who could possibly do something like that in a yoga studio, right? But by then, students from the next class had already arrived, and instead of helping her, he told her to wait longer, mumbling something about patience. After she excused herself for a while, he was still not done, so she began to wonder if she could go, and she should have, because once he was done, instead of providing an answer to her question, he slammed it. In fact, he shut it down completely in her face.

Here's how and why:

She first told him about the one legged king pigeon pose that she had been taught in a class by another local teacher, and then tried to explain the wonderful variation she recently came up with. She also indicated that it was the only one she'd finally found after many years of terrible pain that actually keeps it at bay all day, and that she had only come to ask if it had a SPECIFIC NAME that she could pass on to all of you. But, instead, he snapped.

Believe it or not, (note that this author has witnesses), instead of providing the name, or any support, aid or appreciation, she got slammed, most likely because he was trying to hide the fact that he did not know the answer in front of other students. Immediately, like a "kill joy," he silenced her altruistic query, verbally slapped her in the face, and nailed her coffin shut by barking, "don't do that."

Amazing!

Surprised, hurt down to her soul, and appalled at his sheer gall and audacity, it took a while for this author to get over the shock. But, later that day, it occurred to her that she could do wonders with this story, turning that lemon into lemonade. Here goes:

First, she enjoyed giving him a "name," which is so fair because that's what he refused to do for all of you. It's the title of this specific section, "snarl" which is tailor-made, a perfect fit, because it captures his real name (which will remain nameless, right?), exactly what he did, and his "personality," that is, total lack of one.

But, it is also the perfect segue for this secret chapter. Here's why:

B. Silence, Solitude

It is undisputable that although God is everywhere, the best place to find Him is within silence, while meditating alone in solitude. The same is very true for healing yoga poses and its nirvana bliss.

C. Taking Time

Even just on physical and emotional levels, the release of pain pockets could take time. Rushing would be foolish. One may not be able to keep pace with other class students, which would also be a selfish disservice to them, who'd have to wait for you.

D. Coaxed Out of Hiding

Yet, the most helpful pose or God might NOT want an audience. Either might instead need to be coaxed out of hiding, not because of shyness, but to be most beneficial for YOU.

E. Let the Spirit Move You

These days, freestyle "spirit dancing," so free that it might not even keep to the beat at all, is quite popular. It's also called "trance dancing," akin to other, ancient and even foreign practices known as "swirling dervishes." The idea is total abandon—what a feeling, being swept up by the music into the dance, so much that one might go past sweet bliss and have a total out-of-body experience.

In fact, this author has recently read articles in published yoga magazines in which teachers instruct their students to take their yoga practice beyond, by letting "it" move them. Most students may have no idea what that means, and feel subconscious when it doesn't immediately happen amongst others during a class. That could have a detrimental effect of future deterrence.

Thus, the best place to let the spirit move you is in secret.

F. "Don't Do That" Disclaimer

On the other hand, if no one is present to watch and guide, there could be potential danger, so the best way to turn the "snarl" into lemonade is to use it to point out this disclaimer—do this ONLY at your OWN risk. Results will be on the doer, NOT this book's author, exactly because of this integrated, express, written, recorded statement.

G. Do What Feels Best

Search your heart and soul, and then do what you feel is best. At first, you may want to practice alone with only a book, or the opposite, in a basic class with others. Similarly, to let the spirit move you into awesome pose variations, do that alone or where someone could watch you—you be the judge--decide for yourself.

H. Gut/God/Grace

When your head contradicts your heart, making a good decision may seem impossible, so trust yourself, that is, your gut feeling, because once that "muscle" is developed, it has a secret silver lining—it IS grace and God, speaking to you in secret.

I. Play Cat and Mouse

Since we all have free will, God can't just come out and tell us what to do. And, if He told us too quick, it would be "game over". Life is meant to be a slow dance, yet also a fun-filled adventure, a game of cat and mouse, constantly illusive. One must learn to play, to love the journey, not the destination.

Why?

J. The Secret Secret

Because the secret, secret is that YOU, yourself are God, His golden child, playing with Yourself, and it would not be fun if you found out too quickly. How much fun was it to find out that there is no Santa Clause---right? Wasn't that worth the wait? But, this includes the opposite, as well. Once the masks are off, and true identities are revealed, as Shakespeare said, "all the world is a stage...," so you get to play many more roles than before. Specifically, once the secret, secret is out, there's no one stopping you, no one in your way blocking your flight path to total bliss.

K. Bliss, Remiss

You ARE that bliss, albeit remiss. No one may have ever told you.

L. Go For It!

But, now that you do know, go for it, and do it for yourself, by yourself, with others or not—you decide, take it as far as you wish.

M. Go for the Gold!

Don't settle for anything less—go for the gold. As the following picture demonstrates, there are many ways to play.

In it, the cat is either playing with, or catching, the mouse as it multi-tasks, while it's also enjoying doing yoga, like a synchronized swimmer, with its owner. So cute and sweet!

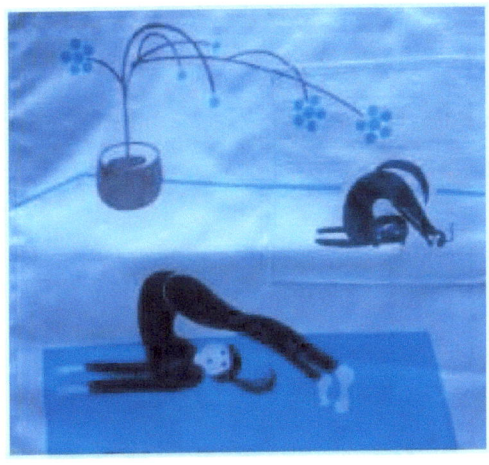

N. Soar More

Bottom line: Get more out of yoga—the sky's the limit!

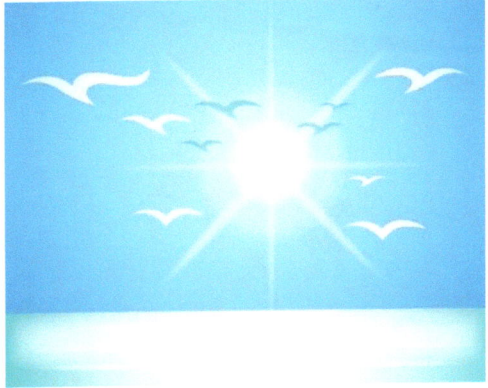

ENDNOTES

A. Error Apology

As always, this author apologizes for any errors, type-os, etc.

B. No Page Numbers

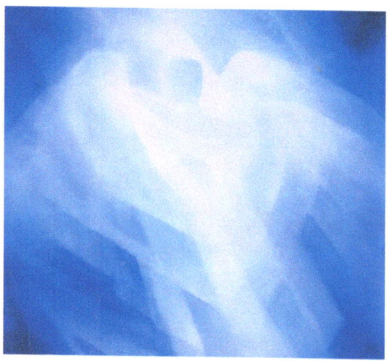

Page numbers were purposefully deleted to impart the feeling of the Holy Spirit soaring this up to the sky, leaving no footprints or evidence at all, as Jesus might in the sand when He carries us.

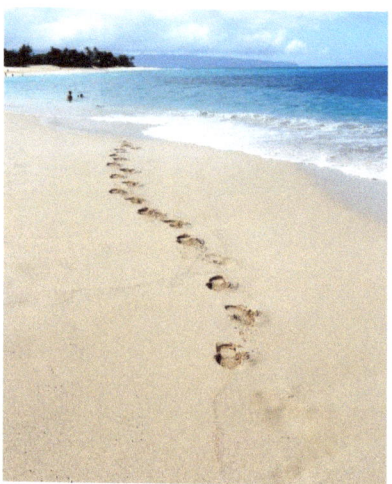

ABOUT THE AUTHOR

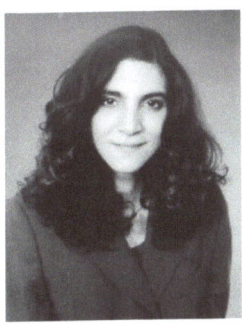 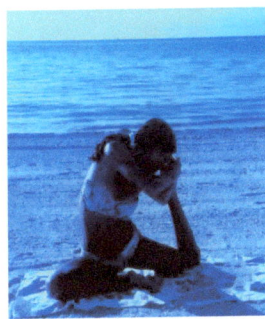

Maryann Fenicato, Esq., Ph.D., was born in Pittsburgh, PA, USA. From highly-accredited Duquesne University, she earned 2 separate doctorates in Law and Philosophy (Ethics), and 3 other degrees.

<u>Currently</u>: To her, yoga is like a salvation, a life-long true LOVE. Sharing, caring and extolling its limitless possibilities, she is a fun, charismatic, motivational, inspirational and educational speaker, teacher, guru, mentor and life coach, who travels domestically and abroad to speak in front of large groups at universities, colleges and other educational institutions, churches, youth facilities and other spiritual organizations, businesses and corporations. Yet, she also enjoys privately counselling individuals confidentially, especially troubled teens or adults who have yet to maximize their destined potential, inspiring God-centered, dream-achieved lives! A former corporate litigation paralegal, peaceful yet court-victorious attorney, cool university professor who won two "Outstanding Professor of the Year Awards" at PITT, and prolific author (far beyond all of her recently published sweet freelance books, her prior legal and philosophical publication titles, alone, form a book much, much bigger than this!), she's already accomplished an amazing destiny. After taking a huge leap of faith to retire and/or walk away from both structured and limited careers, she's now living life to the fullest, the one she'd always dreamed of., in beautiful Key West! So, she enjoys sharing and showing others how to do it, too. For any such engagements, contact: **mafenicato@hotmail.com**

See also her website: **http://maryannfenicato.com**

www.ingramcontent.com/pod-product-compliance
Lightning Source LLC
Chambersburg PA
CBHW050911290526
45792CB00002B/767